ULTIMATE KETO DIET GUIDE

Table of Contents

INTRODUCTION

Keto diets work by glucose, like most low-carb diets. Since many people live on a high-carb diet, our bodies keep running on glucose (or sugar) always for their strength. We can't influence glucose and bring in 24 hours of interest in the tissue and liver of our muscles. When glucose is never accessible again from sources of sustenance, then we start to eat put away fat and fat from our food.

In this way, if you adopt a ketogenic diet program for tenderness, the body absorbs fat as opposed to starches, so many people quickly shed pounds and excess muscles to fat, while they consume fatty bunches and enough calories during their day-to-day food consumption. Another favored critique of the keto diet is that there is no persuasive reason to regulate calories, eat, and attempt to consume a large amount of excellent exercise.

It is all like the Atkins diet, which almost allows the body to eat the expendable fat in just low-carbon products, discarding foods high in carbohydrates and sugar. Out of starch, sustenance fructose causes the body to consume fat for energy. The main differences between exemplary Keto and Atkins diet are that formerly healthier Keto fats are emphasized, less by abundant protein, and no handled meat (e.g., bacon) while further research is being conducted to improve their adequacy.

Such discrepancies with Atkins trace a portion of the traditional dietary myths, such as another high-protein plan that prescribes fat and which hardly any science can figure out what benefits are. These are simple and straightforward nutritional lies.

The keto diet is sound? Is it Atkins's style done? No. No. In any case, if sound fats, greens, and natural meats are appropriate?

CHAPTER ONE

HOW ARE YOU GOING INTO KETOSIS?

People usually asked if keto diet works? However, you can only get your body ketosis off the street. This is how you get your body into ketosis and begin to consume fat to fuel for students in a keto diet: the use of sugar glucose — grains, vegetables that are wearable, a single item, etc.— is cut down by the course of action.

It leads the body to seek an additional source of fuel: fat (think avocados, coconut oil, salmon).

Whereas, without glucose, the body begins to grow fat and develops ketones in the same way.

When the ketone levels in the blood increase to a stage, you are ketosis.

A high ketone disorder results in a fast and healthy weight loss until the bodyweight is high and stable.

Do you care about how many carbohydrates you can eat and are still "in ketosis?" In the standard ketogenic diet for those with epilepsy, about 75% of calories were obtained from big wells (for example, oils or fatty cuts in meat), 5% from starches, and 20% from protein. For many people, a less drastic modification (what I call a "modified keto diet") will help to safely and often rapidly reduce weight.

To adjust and remain in this country, the recommended calculation of total carbs usually amounts to around 30 to 50 net grams. This is seen as an increasingly moderate or adaptable form, but can in the first place, be less overwhelming. If you're acclimatized continuously to "eating keto," you can take carbs down much more if you want (perhaps only occasionally) to about 20 grams of net carbohydrates daily. This is known as the normal, "exact" amount most keto-dieters expect to keep for the best results but note that everyone is slightly different.

Step by step guidance on how to start the Keto Diet plan Proper ratios of the recommended macronutrients (or your macros) will correlate with your current health and well-being day after day (grams of carbs versus fat versus protein). Your age, gender, action aspect, and current body synthesis may also decide on your carbohydrates versus your fat.

For, a keto diet is limited to sugar intake of just 20–30 net grams per day. Net carbs are the indicator of the remaining carbs if dietary fibers are included. Because tissues are toxic when ingested, the vast majority do not count grams of fiber daily.

As such, whole carbs–fiber grams= net carbs. This is the carb controls that matter most.

In the case of a„ severe "(standard) keto diet, fats normally produce around 70 to 80% of the total calories for daily use, protein about 15 to 20%, and sugar only about 5%. In any case, a liberal "fair" way of dealing with keto is also a decent alternative for some people that can take into consideration a more straightforward transition into incredibly low-carbon consumption and improved adaptability (more on these kinds of plans below).

What can you eat on a keto diet? Guidelines on how to make the keto diet with little regard to the structure that you follow: 1. Don't load protein Something that doesn't make the keto diet the same as other low-carb diets are not "protein-loading." Protein isn't as plentiful a part of the keto diet as fat appears. Reason: the body can change protein into glucose in small amounts, which means if you eat lots of it, especially when arranging first, it will impede the progress of your body to ketosis.

The consumption of proteins should be between one and 1.5 grams per kilogram of your total body weight. Separate your optimal load by 2.2 to switch pounds to kilograms. A lady weighing 150 pounds (68 kilograms) should, for example, get about 68–102 grams of protein daily.

2. Track your macros are your meat, protein, and net carbs (not to be confused with calories!). It can be difficult to monitor your macros and your net carbs, so I encourage you to download a keto program that includes a diet that connects your computer.

3. Please consider using some keto supplements for more notable accomplishments Exogenous ketones (prevalently called keto diet pills) are an excellent keto medication that can allow you to achieve results while you reside in this country. (Don't mistake exogenous ketones for raspberry ketones as the latter don't take ketones into the body, or duplicate endogenous ketone in the routine to prevent the use of raspberry ketone.) Also, consider improving the use of amino acid leucine, which is legally divided into acetyl-CoA, making it one of the essential ketogenic amino. While most other amino acids are processed in glucose, leucine-formed acetyl-CoA can be used to produce ketone bodies. It is also present in well-disposed foods such as eggs and curds.

4. Drink water! Drink water!

It is also necessary to drink loads of water, the most essential of all keto beverages. Having enough water helps to prevent your ability from being drained, is vital for processing and helps to conceal. It is also good for detoxification— aiming to drink 10–12 eight-ounce glasses a day.

5. In the end, don't skip days and don't deceive food on a keto diet! Why?! Why? Since a supper with many awful carbs would immediately eliminate you from ketosis and bring you back at the beginning.

When you capitulate and enjoy a cheat meal, anticipate the arrival of some signs of keto influenza... be further consoled by the fact that if you get ketosis now, the body is almost sure to come back soon, and even more quickly than it was initially.

NINE TYPES OF KETO DIET

What's the keto diet again? Moreover, is the keto diet protected and reliable? This available and various types and keto festival plans are usually established with a menu, so to some degree, the answer to the two questions depends on what type of ketogenic plan you are attempting. Currently, we're in nine kinds of the keto diet!

Does it look at how many carbohydrates you can consume and stay "in ketosis?" The standard ketogenic dinner program for epilepsy and its rates of macronutrients are exacting. There are also several types of keto diet models.

These are the basic types of keto diets: the standard ketogenic diet (SKD): the calorie from fat wells (for example, oils or fattier meat cuts), 5% from sugars, and 20% of protein.

The adjusted ketogenic diet (MKD): this supper plan reduces starches to 30 percent of their total calorie intake, with fat and protein expanding separately to 40 and 30 percent.

The CKD: If you feel it is challenging to stick to a low carb diet every day, especially for a long time, you should consider a carbohydrate diet. Carb cycling builds the entry of starch (and calorie occasionally) at the perfect time and in the right amounts, for the most part about 1–2 times per week (for example, at the end of a week).

The guided ketogenic diet (TKD): This eating scheme guides you through the keto diet, but you can add carbohydrates during workouts. So you're going to eat sugar if you work out.

The Confined Ketogenic Diet (CKD): This ketogenic dinner diet was designed to treat diabetes, reduce calories as well as starches. Some studies have shown that limited calories and ketosis can help to manage cancer growth.

A high protein ketogenic diet (PKD), which is frequently used by individuals who must save their bulk like jocks and more established people. In contrast to the protein that makes up 20 percent of food, it is 30 percent. Then, fat falls to 65% of food and carbohydrates stay at 5%. (Alert: kidney issues people shouldn't get the protein to an extreme.) The fan of Veggie's ketogenic diet or a vegan diet: Yes, both can be pictured. Instead of animals, most low carbon, dense veggie lovers, and vegan sustenance are included. Nuts, seeds, low-carbon soil products, greenery, healthy fats, and renewed nutrition are all excellent decisions about a vegetable keto diet. The estuarian system blends keto with veggie fans, dairy as well as pesticide diets, to the degree that everyone recognizes more special health benefits.

Messy keto diet:' Filthiness' is the right term because this type of keto has a precise equivalent amount (75/20/5 of fat/protein/carbs) but instead of concentrating on robust variants of fat such as coconut oil and salmon, a mischievous but cowardly material, such as bacon, Vienna, pork, soft foods, and even cheap keto foods are permitted to consume. I don't say that. I don't recommend this.

The Lazy keto diet gets mistook very often for filthy keto... they are different as the' lethargic' refers to just not following the fat and protein macros (or calories) cautiously. In the meantime, the one view that remaining parts are demanding? Don't eat more than 20 net carb grams a day. A few people discover this shapeless terror, starting or ending with... but I advise that your findings are less critical.

8 EASY MEAL PREP TIPS FOR BEGINNERS

1. Have containers right.

I love glass and silicone containers from BBQ, refrigerator, tender to microwave. Stop dissolving or turning shoddy plastics in a microwave and ensure that whatever you use is durable and hermetically sealed.

Therefore, the procurement of outstanding containers for goods, despite all the problems, is 100% justified because your greens will stay green for much more. These containers increase the airflow of vegetables so that they do not spoil as quickly. Try not to look like my mother and keep food in washed-out containers; it's a significant spill that's close.

2. Keep prepared fixings in advance that you can reliably repurpose in different ways.

Goulash is exceptional, but it can be just one thing very well: a pan. Plan proteins, veggies, and starches should only be a part of your meal preparation schedule as you can repurpose those foods into a few distinct dinners. For example, in portions of mixed greens, in burritos and tacos, in eggs, the pot of simple chipotle dark beans may be used as a side blending with grain and dried vegetables or as the base for a cup. In a sandwich, you can use a cooked chicken bosom platter, a vegetable, and a primary starch protein, for pasta, a snappy soup with chicken stock, noodles and vegetables, destroyed and combined with the BBQ sauce... you get the idea.

3. Two proteins, four vegetables, and one starch follow this equation.

I usually recommend the preparation of two proteins each week, and one of them is meatless so that you can consume more vegetables. Marinated tofu or a mixed green bean plate are two of my best choices. Then prepare some four crops, including a diverse green pot, cut raw vegetables, and fry vegetables. To round off stuff, make a substantial cluster of lonely starch such as fried potatoes or whole grains.

4. See your schedule.

If individuals don't review their schedules before planning a food pack and then take on a wide range of pre-booked activities that they didn't understand they had that week, a part of their team will likely go into the wastepaper. It's a simple fix: don't waste food! Continuously review your schedule before you shop for food and adjust the amount of food you make for any meals you will not need.

5. Get smarter about the health of food.

No one wants to get sick if they try to get music! In all cases, these are corrupt practices when you deal with meat. Nonetheless, they are particularly important when preparing your dinner because you will make substantial food clusters and place them on more extended periods, which raises the danger of foodborne illness.

Default #1: Do not give up a large cluster of anything to chill out in a large tray on the oven, stove, or refrigerator. You need to cool quickly so that the food is partitioned into small containers and put into the more relaxed or more comfortable. Remember, bottles of name and date.

Principle #2: Cook food at the right time. As demonstrated by the United States Agriculture Division and U.S. Food and Drug Administration, meat and fish, depending on the kind of food, should be cooked at between 145 degrees Fahrenheit and 165 degrees. (Look on the foodsafety.gov chart for points of interest.) Invest for simple temperature readings in food thermometers (in general, approximately $5 to $15).

Guideline #3: Maintain raw and cooked food free from expected sullying. I think you know this, but it's just a recommendation to wash your hands and make surfaces when handling raw foods, eggs, fish, and other food.

Standard #4: The majority of remains remain in the icebox for 3 to 4 days. Look for more detail in these guidelines. When you are hot scraps, make sure they hit a Fahrenheit of 165 degrees and offer nothing chance to sit for more than 2 hours at temperatures of 40 ° C to 140 ° C as microbes will easily double inside this temperature sprint.

6. Cook a few accessories on a single sheet pan.

In the event you expect that you can prepare most of your proteins, starches, and vegetables at the same time (who wouldn't want to spend some time contemplating these things?), one-off dinners are great. Some of my favas are this spirited garlic tofu plate, and Brussels grows, sesame tofu and vegetables, these vegetarian and meat burrito bowls and the brie apple and flawless chicken bosom.

I put most of my vegetables into olive oil and salt, spread them on the protein plate, and cook everything together. So basic. So basic.

7. Use sauces, spices, and marinades to fluctuate your suppers and to prevent similar fixations from becoming exhausted.

Select a supporter for the sound is the season and build your basic dinner around it. Along these lines, you have the taste of assembling the meal. Take a pesto purchased locally, hurl cherry tomatoes and chicken bosoms, for example, and eat in the stove: one skillet, three attachments. Over. Done. Another suggestion is to use miso as a snappy marinade for the flank steak, sear it at that point with scallions and Buk Choy, or Thai curry glue with a little fish before you grill it with greens. I always keep baked rice, tahini, dark beans, and garlic sauce in my kitchen for purity!

8. Pre-prepared attachments are an incredibly easy route.

There's nothing wrong with taking one or two accessible routes. For example, rotisserie chicken is an excellent supermarket prepared food that people seem to love the most. All things considered: When else would you say that you are most likely to eat whole chicken grilled again without staying close for an hour to cook first? Expel the hair, shaker, and throw in mixed green plates or use in such recipes as my chicken enchiladas.

CHAPTER TWO

THE BEGINNER'S GUIDE TO MEAL PREP

The most effective method of preparing food for several days at the same time might seem to be a fantastic challenge. In any case, once you get it, it's straightforward. Here's a handbook for the start.

1. Rigging up. Rigging up.

Given what some supper planning aids can suggest before you begin, you don't have to spend large amounts of new products. It can be quite helpful to have the right phones. Try keeping these things if you haven't got them now.

A few large skillets. Use them for cooking vegetables, proteins, or full sliced foods.

A big stockpot. For one-pot foods like soups, stews, curry, or bean stew, this is vital.

A small pan of sauce. Use it for cooking whole grains or for growing hard-bubbled eggs.

Sustainable glass storage compartments. These are the best choices to bring prepared food away. (They won't leak chemical substances into your diet in comparison to plastic, too.) Look for having a variety of sizes for throwing out clumps of prepared items of all shapes and sizes.

Packs of Zip-tops. Kids are exceptional for dividing bites such as nuts or cut veggies. Greater ones help hold whole meals or individual parts when you are short of storage shelves (or are out of space for more holders in your ice chest).

2. Plan your schedule. Prepare your meal.

You must make sense of what you are going to do before you start cooking. The combination helps you to remain satisfied with meat, vegetable, and starch for each dinner. The sky is the cutoff, though in general, the best supper prepares meals can be categorized as one of these classifications: one-pot or one-container meals: soups, curry, beans, and cereals, or whatever else you can prepare in a separate pot or Crock-Pot. "These are an excellent choice in particular because you don't have to apply anything but condiments to the feast," f. Sheet meals and frittatas (heat them to a large bowl and cut them into cuts or render portions in biscuit tins) are also used here. If you want simplicity to the utmost, this is the way to go.

Part-based meals: do you want something more? Have a go at the preparation and organization solely of proteins, vegetables, and starches. Pre-hacked plants can, for example, top a pizza on Mondays, be put in pasta sauce on Tuesdays, and collapse into tacos on Wednesdays. However, as a simple bowl of quinoa, vegetables, and chicken can become exhaustive, they intend to prepare a few sauces, dressings, or garnishes to make things interesting from flavors.

Do you have to describe all you'll eat all week? Not a chance. "To plan most meals can work for specific individuals. But, it's vital, especially when you start to have dinner prepared, that you start a small start. So, if managing five or even seven days seems like an excessive amount, make two dinners. Double the fixtures so that you can have two suppers every time, and bam! You have four night free. (These equations take a short approach!) Cook vegetables and eat chicken or tofu, when you start the stove. A pot of quinoa or soup begins at that point on the stovetop. She proposes stewing, pre-slashing natural products or veggies, or preparing a cluster of hummuses for nibbling.

4. Pack it up. Pack it up.

Did you have all your food prepared? All done! Well done! It's an excellent chance to store everything, so you'll have easy access to your meals and fixtures. Three critical reminders: use the right compartments. Divide single pieces into small individual owners, which are hard to get and go. Meals that you prepare in a significant group can be delivered in higher areas.

Maintain parts of mixed greens and clothes discreet. A solution for muddy, withered rubble is to remove dressed servings of mixed greens effectively. Hold all fresh by pressing in one holder the cleaved plate of mixed green veggies, dress in another.

Heat before heating. It is good to replace the hot food directly with your glass storage vessels. Provide the food with the opportunity to get to room temperature before it is transferred to the ice chest–especially about large clumps. Popping into the more relaxed, a family-sized service of a sizzling bean stew will heat everything that is already there. This could imaginably set the stage for decay and unhealthy nutrition.

5. Cook deliberately.

You have this delicious food to eat–what is it recommended that you eat first? In any case, creature-based proteins will usually lose their shine the snappiest. But consider eating meat before a week and avoiding plant-setting proteins later, as Jones prescribes. It's dependable to use your intuition if something looks or scents. "Many foods can be set up before time and remain safe to eat for five days.

EFFORTLESS KETO MEAL PREP

If you at any point figured you could depend on motivation to get more fit (or structure any sound propensity), you most likely understood this system is worthless. It's not merely you — nobody can keep up unshakeable motivation always. Research indicates arranging altogether improves your probability of progress contrasted with motivation alone. The report demonstrated that 91% of members who booked exercise worked out in any event once every week. Just 35% of the gathering that didn't plan it is working out at any rate once per week. When you need some persuading, here are three additional motivations to begin meal preparing immediately.

#1: Meal Prep Conquers Decision Fatigue

Choice fatigue is the motivation behind why individuals like Obama wear similar garments each day. We people have restricted willpower, and the more choices we need to make, the more uncertain we are to make the correct one. Scientists broke down 1,100 choices to discharge detainees on parole made by judges through the span of a year. Detainees who seemed promptly toward the beginning of the day got probation around 70 percent of the time, while the individuals who seemed late in the day were paroled under 10 percent of the time. "

The parole choice had next to no to do with the wrongdoing or conditions and undeniably more to do with the number of options the judge recently made that day.

Much the same as with the judge, each little choice you make diminishes your willpower. When your meal plan, you lessen the measure of decisions you need to make about what to eat every day, expelling willpower from the condition.

#2: Meal Prep Help You Save Time and Money

If you can concentrate on food for several hours out of each week, shopping, baking, and preparing meals are endless hours in the week.

#3: Meal Prep Can Help You Achieve Ketosis

One of the most important things to keep to the ketogenic diet is your macros. You have a better opportunity to do your job.complete goals by adopting a keto-friendly meal plan. What are you able to eat on a ketogenic diet? Improve flexibility with Burn Fat Secrets.

What are you able to eat in a ketogenic diet?

A ketogenic diet is generally an eating routine that changes from expending sugar to consuming fat across your organism. About 99 percent of the global population have some sugar-conserving meat. In this way, sugars are the primary source of fuel used in the preparation of carbs. This technique makes weighty people. Anyway, a fat and ketone diet will cause weight adversity. As you are asking what you can eat on a ketogenic diet, you eat up to 30-50 grams of carbohydrate consistently. Next, let us logically find out what you can get on your plate and how your ketogenic diet affects your growth.

IMPORTANCE OF THE KETOGENIC DIET SUGAR CAUTION

When you enter the bloodstream after storage, the body moves from a carbohydrate burner to a fat, these carbohydrates include the vital sugar known as glucose. The body can accumulate such a large amount of glucose before dumping it somewhere else. An overabundance of glucose leads to the so-called fat in the intestine, cushy layers and so on.

Protein and Its Place in Keto

Protein is a source of sugar that a couple of people ignore in their eating routine. Protein over-consumption by measuring your body obstruction will result in weight gain. Since our body changes into sugar over excess protein, we should coordinate the amount of protein we eat. Control of our protein confirmation is a bit like eating ketogenic and getting slimmer. Most importantly, recognize your opposition to protein step by step and use it as a manual to confirm the enhancement perfectly. Secondly, choose your protein, for example, naturally, keep free eggs and grass meats. Finally, make dinners in an enjoyable group and keep your energy for the food routine. For example, a five-ounce steak and a few eggs can give specific individuals the ideal daily protein proportion.

Caloric Intake on the Ketogenic Diet

Calories are another significant idea about what you could consume in a ketogenic diet. The quality of the calories we spend on food helps the body stay healthy. We should, therefore, eat enough calories to satisfy our everyday wholesome requirements. Calories are a weight for some people who use different diets. As a ketogenic dietitian, you don't have to fear calorie tallying so much. Most people on a low-carb diet eat 1500–1700 kcals per day in calories.

Fats, The Good and The Bad

Protein does not occur in many high-sound fats, like nuts, seeds or olive oil, in whole foods healthy fats form a key component of the ketogenic diet and can be created in breaks, tidbits or attachments. Misinterpretations of food protein are that a high proportion of them are irritating and cause weight gain. Although the two clarifications are true, the fat which we consume is not the fast explanation of the fat which exists on our skin. Or perhaps, on the other side, the sugar from each change we invest is the thing that finally becomes fat in our collection.

Equalization Your Nutrients Wisely

Absorption leads to sugars that we eat in the bloodstream and the amount of abundance moves into our fatty cells. Low starch and low protein consumption result in a wealth of body fat as such foods contain sugar. Unreasonable intake of any food is therefore undesirable and contributes to weight gain. A solid diet includes parity of protein, sugars, and fats as the dimensions of the resilience of your body indicate.

Almost everyone can follow a ketogenic diet with enough commitment and effort. Besides, we can typically guide specific significant conditions with keto. Insulin blockage, increased blood sugar, inflammation, obesity, Type 2 diabetes are a few welfare conditions that may be resolved. All these unfavorable conditions will decrease and standardize the injured person who has a solid ketogenic diet. Low-carbon, high-fat and moderate protein foods give this diet its extraordinary medical advantages.

CONCLUSION

For some, the ketogenic diet is a phenomenal catastrophe option. The person on the menu can eat a routine that requires sustenance that you can not predict through and through.

So, the ketogenic diet is an eating regimen of unusually low carbohydrates and high fat. How many meals would you end your day with bacon and eggs, Save them for lunch and then for dinner, steak and broccoli in line with chicken wings? That might sound unreasonable to some. Ok, this nutrition scheme is a day of cognitive blowing and you tried to meet the expectations perfectly with that festival program.

When you eat a small proportion of carbohydrates, your body is ketosis. This means that your body uses fat for essentiality. How little carbs do you need to consume to get ketosis? It varies from one person to another. In any case, the stone is set to remain under 25 net carbohydrates. Many would recommend that you remain below ten net carbohydrates when you are in "affirmation master" that is where you put your body into ketosis.

Let me support you if you're not sure what net carbs are. Net carbon is the amount of carbon that you consume less than dietary fiber. So, when you eat 35 grams of net carbs and 13 grams of nutritional fiber each day, the net carbs will be 22 per day. Sufficiently clear, right? What else is interesting about Keto, so adjacent weight hardship? Various people think of increased mental concentration in a routine. Another advantageous position has imperative development. This is a decreased need.

9 781699 931882